Surviving a Mud Run

Finishing Spartan, Warrior Mudder, and More!

By: John Rouda

Copyright © 2015 John Rouda

ISBN-10: 1507628137
ISBN-13: 978-1507628133

DEDICATION

To my wife, who taught me that I can always do a little more than my mind says I can. For this, I thank you.

I love you very much.

CONTENTS

CHAPTER 1
BEFORE YOU START

This book is designed to inform you guys about what you're getting into if you've signed up for a mud run of any kind.

I'm neither a great runner nor a fitness professional. **Please consult your physician before starting any workout program**. I'm in no way qualified to write a fitness book, except for the fact that I've done this before. I came from a non-runner background, but I have completed many mud runs over the last ten years. I can give you a unique perspective on how to get it done

The truth of it is, I'm an IT Manager and Computer Science Professor. It may seem pretty strange that I'm writing about mud runs. My last book, *Surviving a 5K Race*, is similar in fashion to this book. It's all about how to start from zero and get through a 5k. We're not going to be starting from zero here. I'm going to assume you're at least capable of completing (now I didn't say running) a 5K race. If not, please refer to my latest book *Surviving a 5K Race.* You can get it by going to http://johnrouda.com/5k/.

My first mud run was the USMC Ultimate Challenge Mud Run in Columbia, SC. I was warned ahead of time that I should plan on throwing away the cloths and shoes that I would be wearing. I did some online research on the obstacles and challenges, but that wasn't enough to fully prepare me for the journey that I was about to take.

Once you start participating in mud runs, be prepared to be hooked. I recently ran a Spartan Race in Charlotte, NC with a group of coworkers. One of the runners was participating in his first mud run. He went on to do four more that year and we ran the Spartan Race again in Charlotte the following year. What I'm trying to say is that running mud runs can be highly addictive. Okay, you've been warned. Let's proceed.

Before you start following this or any other running guide, let me lay down some ground rules to help you succeed.

You're Running Shoes
I recommended in *Surviving a 5k Race* that everyone get fitted for running shoes. Here is why you should do that before you start training.

I skipped this step at first and started running in the same shoes that I wore when I played tennis, played basketball, cut the grass... that was a big mistake. After a few weeks, I started getting knee pain and found that my shoes were starting to cause a mild case of runner's knee. I decided to get fitted at a local store in Charlotte, NC. They watched me run (without shoes) and took a close look at my feet using some special tools. Then they said I needed firm support and recommended some super expensive Saucony running shoes. They charged me about $129.99. I now buy the same shoes online for around $60.

Getting fitted for running shoes is well worth the extra money. It helps prevent injuries that typically lead to people feeling like their bodies weren't designed for running. The shoes that you wear when you do your mud run should be older versions of the shoes you train in. Remember, you'll likely want to throw these away after the race.

Don't rush it
For most of you, these workouts and runs

will be new. As with anything that's new, you need to take your time and let your body get used to it. If you just try to go all out on day one, you're likely to be super sore, or worse, get injured. My advice is to take it slow. There's no need to rush.

Pay attention to what you eat and drink
It's important to know that what you put into your body, is what you get out of your body. You need to eat food that your body can convert to energy and use to build muscle when starting any training program, especially one that burns as many calories as burpees. What's a burpee you ask? Oh just wait, it will become either your best friend or worst enemy ☺.

This is the part where I have to stress the importance of water. Not sodas and sports drinks-- water. Have a drink of water the night before you run, right before you workout, when you wake up, before bed, and, of course, after you've completed a workout. Stay hydrated. Your body is mostly water. Keep it that way.

Get motivated

I'm on a kick about motivation right now. I've been watching all the Ted Talks and reading all the books I can find on motivation. Daniel Pink's book, *Drive*, is a great resource on how to motivate people and I want to take some of those concepts into account when talking about working out and preparing for a race. In his book, Pink talks about using Autonomy, Mastery, and Purpose for your motivation. Here's how I apply those to running a mud run:

- **Autonomy:** Remember that we are free to run and workout. We're not living in a society where we're bound from these luxuries. We "get to" workout; we don't "have to" workout. If you keep that mindset, it makes doing the routines and runs much easier.

- **Mastery:** Mastery is all about self-improvement. We're not looking for perfection here, just progress. Peter Drucker said that "if you can't measure it, you can't improve it." You need to keep track of your reps, sets, run times, etc. If you do that, you'll see improvement and will be motivated to work even harder and survive this mud run.

- **Purpose:** Realize that running this mud run is for more than just you. If you have a family, getting in shape will help you live longer. Also most races donate or support charitable organizations, so remember that you're supporting a cause. Let that keep you motivated.

Find a Race

The next thing you need to do before continuing this book is find a race. Look for one about six to eight weeks out so that you can start training today. Not tomorrow, not next week, not next month. Today. As my wife will attest, if you're like me and like to put something off until tomorrow, you might as well put it off forever. If you're reading this book because you already have a race and it's less than eight weeks away, then you better get started!

CHAPTER 2

THE EXERCISES

In this chapter, we'll go over the essential exercises that you'll need to know in order to prepare for a mud run. Remember that most mud runs are not just nice runs through mud. They include scaling walls, climbing ropes, dragging weights, flipping tires, crawling under barbed wire, and much more. These exercises will help get your body where it needs to be to endure the punishment that it will go through. If you're up for the challenge, read on.

Pull-ups

Imagine having to pull yourself out of knee-deep mud in order to climb up to the next obstacle, or having to climb up and over a wall. A pull-up is the best exercise to train for those particular situations. This exercise fully engages the back and bicep muscles. Pull-ups are the most important exercise to do as you prepare for a mud run. You can get a pull bar to attach to your door. To see the one that I use and recommend, visit http://runbikehike.us/mudrun/

Push-ups

The best bodyweight exercise (in my opinion) is push-ups. Do you know why? They are effective regardless of the physical endeavor you are striving for. In this case, push-ups will help improve upper body strength and overall endurance. While most people wouldn't make that correlation between push-ups and mud runs, it is a match made in heaven. Think about it. Who do you think will climb walls quicker, someone with the ability of doing fifty push-ups or ten push-ups? I rest my case.

Squats
While push-ups are the best bodyweight exercise for the upper body, squats are the most fundamental exercise for the lower body. I actually hate squats, but they work so well I can't write this book without them. It's impossible to get through these challenging mud races without strong, durable legs. By doing squats, you will build strength and endurance in all your major lower body muscles: glutes, hamstrings, quads and calves. Last time I checked, all of those muscle groups will be greatly needed as you embark on a mud run.

Sprints
Quick question: How can you get better at racing without running? Maybe I should have said, "trick question," because you can't. To improve in any endeavor, you have

to actually practice doing that endeavor. Sprints will greatly aid your ability to compete in a mud run. Sprints will help improve endurance levels as well as burn body fat that would weigh you down. Sprints help build strong legs as well. So whether you're on an Olympic track, your driveway, or on a treadmill, sprints can and should be performed.

Bent Over Rows
If pull-ups are too difficult, then bent over rows should be a part of your exercise arsenal. Even if pull-ups aren't too difficult, you can still get great value from bent over rows. You can do these with free weights or with bands. To see the bands that I use when training for my mud runs, visit http://runbikehike.us/mudrun. Bent over rows will not only help build a strong back and arms, they will balance the strength within your back. A strong back is essential to prepare for all of the crawling, climbing, and pulling that you will likely do at a mud

run race.

Burpees

Love them or hate them-- burpees are a must. If you can't complete an obstacle during a Spartan Race, guess what you have to do to move on: thirty burpees. If you need an effective total body exercise to quickly improve endurance, burpees should be your exercise of choice. This exercise was popularized when the United States Armed Services adopted it as a way to assess the fitness level of recruits during WWII. Burpees combine squats and push-ups to deliver a heart-pounding, muscle-building movement that will leave you gasping for breath. Burpees will have you mud race ready in no time. In my opinion, if you're tackling the Spartan Race or Tough Mudder, this is the exercise of choice.

Run up a Hill

One of the best ways to get mud race ready is to practice running up hills. Most obstacle courses will have a hill, or several, that you have to climb. If not prepared, your calves will hate you with a passion. Your entire lower body will be worked fully from doing a couple intervals of hill runs. If you're out of shape, start out walking up the hill then progress to jogging, running, and then sprinting.

Bear Crawls
Walking like a bear will help you get ready for a mud run. Bear crawls are an excellent exercise that will build overall musculature (especially shoulders, stomach and legs) while improving endurance levels. Many of the courses will have obstacles where you have to climb through mud under barbed wire. Bear crawls will prepare you for that.

Chair Dips
Most people don't know that 2/3 of their arm muscles are their triceps, not their biceps. In my opinion, chair dips are the most effective at-home exercise for building

and strengthening your triceps. You can do these anytime and anywhere, even at work.

Mountain Climbers

No, you won't be climbing up a mountain, but it will feel like you have when you do this exercise right. Mountain climbers will prepare you for climbing obstacle courses. This is a great exercise to use to burn fat, build muscle, and boost endurance levels. It may not be as tough as climbing a mountain, but it will help prepare you for climbing at a mud race.

Side Hops (also called Lateral Hops)

Besides being a perfect exercise to use in order to dodge your spouse when they are getting on your nerves, it will help prepare you for a mud race. It practically targets every muscle below your waist and burns a lot of calories while building muscular legs. In case you're in a mud run that involves dodge ball, this movement will have you ready.

Running

You didn't think you'd get off without running, did you? As I stated earlier, you need to be in 5K shape to consider a sprint class mud run. If you want to do a longer one, be sure you can run the distance. Some Spartan Races and Tough Mudders are 12 miles long or longer. You have to be able to run that far in order to finish the race, so be sure to train running the distance of your race or further. If you're not in 5K shape, check out *Surviving a 5K Race* at http://johnrouda.com/5k/.

The Burpee Run

I saved the best exercise for last. Remember that you have to do thirty burpees if you can't complete an obstacle in a Spartan Race. Having run a few mud runs in the past, I know how hard it is to do physically tough activities right after a run and, conversely, how hard it is to run right after doing physically tough activities. To help with this, I created the burpee run. A burpee run is really simple. It's just a run (you choose the distance) with thirty burpees every quarter or half mile, depending on how "hard core" you really are.

Making it a Habit

Now before we get started in the weekly training, let's move into something that I think is really important: habits. I got hooked on *The Power of Habit* by Charles Duhigg. S.J. Scott is another author who has written dozens of books about habits. I'm bringing this up, because when you make exercise a habit, it's so much easier to stick with it instead of putting it off. I wrote about this in my last book, but I think it's important enough to include it here, too.

There are three steps to creating any good habit and three "R's" in the framework for habit change. If you're interested in more about habits, please check out *The Power of Habit* or other habit books on my resources page at http://runbikehike.us/resources.

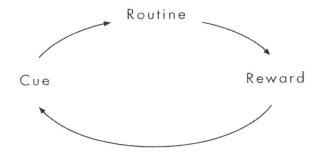

Routine

Cue

Reward

The 3 R's of Habit Change that form a "habit loop":

- **Reminder (Cue)** (The trigger that starts the new behavior): For me, this is the hardest part. I'm so inconsistent when it comes to setting routines. For most people, it's all about timing. Either they run after work, or in the morning before work, or at lunch. However, for me, I found that I would run when I wanted to. I didn't have a specific time set-aside in the morning or evening.

When I was training for the OBX Marathon, getting into the habit of running was really tough. I didn't have a good reminder. After several weeks, I finally got into a pattern of running. Looking back on it, it all happened when I made up my mind to run right after work. This "reminder" triggered my routine and helped me make running a habit.

- **Routine** (The behavior or action you're creating/changing): This is the easy part. Start running. Your routine schedule is outlined in the following chapters.

- **Reward** (The benefit for the behavior): This if the fun part. Give yourself a reward. For me candy, food, etc. usually works. Most of the time it was ice cream. I'm sure that most health professionals will cringe at reading this, but it's the truth. After a while I found that running itself became a sort of reward. I feel good about myself physically and mentally when I run. I know that you will feel the same way eventually.

3 Steps for creating a new habit:

1. **Set your reminder**– This can be a timing thing, like running in the morning, lunch, or after work.

2. **Follow the plan in the book**– This step is pretty easy. Just follow along.

3. **Choose your reward**– Hopefully the act of running will become your reward, but if you need a little motivation to get started, I recommend sugar free or reduced fat ice cream.

CHAPTER 3
WEEK 1 & 2

So you've got eight weeks till your first mud run. Are you physically and mentally ready for that? Will you easily make it to the finish line or make a mud face (i.e. fall flat on your face in the mud)? How prepared you are will dictate your success. The training guides for week 1 and 2 will make sure you start off on the right foot. If you are ready to "murder" a Tough Mudder race or "spank" a Spartan Race, or Whip a Warrior Dash, then proceed! (Sorry about the corny puns... I'm a nerd).

Running

Don't neglect your running. You'll need to continue running three times a week during this training. No one said this would be easy, but if you follow this schedule and work hard, you will succeed. I recommend two runs of a shorter distance, like maybe three miles. Slowly increase the distance until you can complete the maximum distance on your third run of the week. Start slow and don't overdo it. You've got to save your energy for your workouts. I'd also recommend inserting a burpee run if you're up for it. You'll see them in the training as well.

Training Frequency

You will train four days per week. In this sample training guidelines, the training days at the gym will be on Monday, Tuesday, Thursday, and Friday. Wednesday, Saturday and Sunday are active rest days. Choose whatever four days you have at least 45 minutes to an hour to train.

Week 1 Mud Race Training

Monday Training Routine (Week 1)
Warm-up Routine
(do each exercise in order for 1 minute):
- Jog in place
- Jumping Jacks
- Lunge Walks
- Arm Circles

Exercise Routine:
- Push-ups* - 3x 15-20 reps
- Burpees - 3x 12-15 reps
- Chair Dips - 3x 15-20 reps

Do push-ups on your knees if unable to do regular pushups

Tuesday Training Routine (Week 1)
Warm-up Routine
(do each exercise in order for 1 minute):
- Jog in place
- Jumping Jacks

- Lunge Walks
- Arm Circles

Exercise Routine:
- Pull-ups* - 3x 10 reps
- Bent over Rows - 3x 12-15 reps
- Mountain Climbers - 5 x 30 seconds

Use assisted pull-ups with a chair if unable to do regular pull-ups

Wednesday Training Routine (Week 1)
Walk /jog/ run 5 miles today outside or on a treadmill (inclined).

Thursday Training Routine (Week 1)
Warm-up Routine
(do each exercise in order for 1 minute):
- Jog in place
- Jumping Jacks
- Lunge Walks
- Arm Circles

Exercise Routine:
- Push-ups* - 3x 15-20 reps

- Burpees - 3x 12-15 reps
- Squats - 3x 30 reps

Do push-ups on your knees if unable to do regular pushups

Friday Training Routine (Week 1)
Warm-up Routine

(do each exercise in order for 1 minute):
- Jog in place
- Jumping Jacks
- Lunge Walks
- Arm Circles

Exercise Routine:
- Pull-ups* - 3x 11 reps
- Squats - 3x 30 reps
- Mountain Climbers - 3x 30 seconds

Use assisted pull-ups with a chair if unable to do regular pull-ups

Saturday Training Routine (Week 1)

Do some 20-30 minute yoga or other physical activities to help soothe your achy muscles. (If you have kids, play outside with

them). Check out the training videos at
http://runbikehike.us/yoga

Sunday Training Routine (Week 1)
Just completely relax. Kick back and watch
TV, play solitaire, or read a good book. Pick a
relaxing hobby. I'd be building an app or
website.

Week 2 Mud Race Training

Monday Training Routine (Week 2)
Warm-up Routine
(do each exercise in order for 1 minute):
- Jog in place
- Jumping Jacks
- Lunge Walks
- Arm Circles

Exercise Routine:
- Push-ups - 3x 15-20 reps
- Lateral Hops* - 3x 15 reps

- Sprints** - 6x 30 seconds

*Completing a hop on both sides counts as 1 rep
**Find a slope hill to run up

Tuesday Training Routine (Week 2)
Warm-up Routine
do each exercise in order for 1 minute):
- Jog in place
- Jumping Jacks
- Lunge Walks
- Arm Circles

Exercise Routine:
- Pull-ups - 3x 12 reps
- Bear Crawls - 3x 20 Yards
- Squats - 3x 30 reps

Wednesday Training Routine (Week 2)
Walk /jog/ run 5 miles today outside or on a treadmill (incline 3).

Thursday Training Routine (Week 2)
Warm-up Routine (do each exercise in order for 1 minute):

- Jog in place
- Jumping Jacks
- Lunge Walks
- Arm Circles

Exercise Routine:
- Push-ups - 3x 15-20 reps
- Lateral Hops* - 3x 12-15 reps
- Sprints** – 6x 30 seconds

*Completing a hop on both sides counts as 1 rep
**Find a slope hill to run up

Friday Training Routine (Week 2)
Warm-up Routine
(do each exercise in order for 1 minute):
- Jog in place
- Jumping Jacks
- Lunge Walks
- Arm Circles

Exercise Routine:
- Pull-ups - 3x 12 reps
- Bear Crawls - 3x 20 Yards
- Squats - 3x 30 reps

Saturday Training Routine (Week 2)
Yoga time. Watch complete one of the free yoga training videos found at http://runbikehike.us/yoga

Sunday Training Routine (Week 2)
Relax time! You deserve to after two weeks of consistent work getting ready for the mud race.

This was the first two weeks training cycle as you prepare for your mud race. As you can see, this routine isn't easy. But if you want to compete to your upmost ability come race day, this routine will get you ready. If you survived weeks 1 and 2, read on....

Chapter 4
Week 3 & 4

If you're reading this chapter, then congratulations! You survived the first two weeks of intense training in preparation for your mud race. Nonetheless, you still have six weeks until doing battle with obstacle courses. Staying focused is essential because the honeymoon period (i.e. being excited about starting a new program) is over. Now it's all about grit and grind.

Hopefully by now you're starting to feel good about all you've accomplished. I mean, take a look back at all you've done in two weeks. You should be super proud of yourself. If you've missed a day or two, it's okay. Keeping moving forward and try not to miss any more.

Getting ready for this mud run is about continually pushing yourself mentally and physically as you inch closer to race day! So are you ready for the Week 3 and 4 training schedules? I hope so, because here they are.

Week 3 Mud Race Training

Monday Training Routine (Week 3)
Warm-up Routine
(do each exercise in order for 1 minute):
- Jog in place
- Jumping Jacks

- Lunge Walks
- Arm Circles

Exercise Routine:
- Push-ups - 3x 15-20 reps
- Squats - 3x 30 reps
- Mountain Climbers - 5x 40 seconds

Tuesday Training Routine (Week 3)
Warm-up Routine
(do each exercise in order for 1 minute):
- Jog in place
- Jumping Jacks
- Lunge Walks
- Arm Circles

Exercise Routine:
- Pull-ups - 4x 8 reps
- Bear Crawls - 3x 20 Yards
- Run up a hill* - 5x 30 seconds reps

Find an open hill or do this on a treadmill (set incline to the highest available)

Wednesday Training Routine (Week 3)

Pick a leisure activity that involves walking for 1 hour (e.g. walk your dog, go the mall, etc.)

Thursday Training Routine (Week 3)
Warm-up Routine
(do each exercise in order for 1 minute):
- Jog in place
- Jumping Jacks
- Lunge Walks
- Arm Circles

Exercise Routine:
- Pull-ups - 4x 9 reps
- Squats - 3x 30 reps
- Mountain Climbers - 5x 40 seconds

Friday Training Routine (Week 3)
Warm-up Routine
(do each exercise in order for 1 minute):
- Jog in place
- Jumping Jacks
- Lunge Walks

- Arm Circles

Exercise Routine:
- Pull-ups - 4x 9 reps
- Squats - 3x 40 reps
- Mountain Climbers - 5x 40 seconds

Saturday Training Routine (Week 3)
Get with friends and play a sport (e.g. basketball, flag football, tennis, etc.). If you don't have any friends, do another yoga video at http://runbikehike.us/yoga/

Sunday Training Routine (Week 3)
Relax and unwind. Catch up on your favorite TV shows.

Week 4 Mud Race Training

Monday Training Routine (Week 4)
Warm-up Routine
(do each exercise in order for 1 minute):

- Jog in place
- Jumping Jacks
- Lunge Walks
- Arm Circles

Exercise Routine:
- Push-ups - 4x 15-20 reps
- Bear Crawls - 3x 30 yards
- Sprints - 5x 20 yards seconds

Tuesday Training Routine (Week 4)
Warm-up Routine
(do each exercise in order for 1 minute):
- Jog in place
- Jumping Jacks
- Lunge Walks
- Arm Circles

Exercise Routine:
- Pull-ups - 4x 10 reps
- Squats - 3x 30 reps
- Burpees - 5x 20 reps

Wednesday Training Routine (Week 4)

Do some yoga. Find the videos at video at http://runbikehike.us/yoga/

Thursday Training Routine (Week 4)
Warm-up Routine

(do each exercise in order for 1 minute):

- Jog in place
- Jumping Jacks
- Lunge Walks
- Arm Circles

Exercise Routine:

- Push-ups - 4x 15-20 reps
- Bear Crawls - 3x 30 Yards
- Sprints - 5x 20 Yards

Friday Training Routine (Week 4)

Warm-up Routine (do each exercise in order for 1 minute):

- Jog in place
- Jumping Jacks
- Lunge Walks

- Arm Circles

Exercise Routine:
- Pull-ups - 4x 10 reps
- Squats - 3x 40 reps
- Burpees - 5x 20 reps

Saturday Training Routine (Week 4)

Find an activity to do with your family members and/or friends (e.g. throwing a Frisbee, playing softball, etc.). If you don't have any friends… go out and make some. Volunteer, visit a church or meet up event and get some friends. If that's not your thing, then do another yoga video at http://runbikehike.us/yoga/.

Sunday Training Routine (Week 4)

Relax! As a matter of fact, go get a massage. You deserve it!

That's it for weeks 3 and 4. If you've already made it through week 4, then you've got one full month finished. Be sure to take some time and celebrate. One of the things that can really help you succeed at your goals is to celebrate small wins. Completing 1 month of this training program is a great accomplishment; celebrate it!

Congrats and get ready for week 5!

CHAPTER 5
WEEK 5 & 6

After one month of putting mud... I mean blood, sweat, and tears... into your mud run training program, you should be feeling pretty frickin' good! If anything, your body should be more adept to handle the stresses of an obstacle course. Nonetheless, you're one month away from your official mud race. More work is needed in order to maximize your chances of success, but the good news is that you're half way there.

I really hope that you've started to see a change in your body and your strength. Depending on your genetics and your diet, you may or may not see a noticeable difference in the mirror, but I bet the exercises are easier. Do more reps if that's true. This is just another sign that you're getting stronger and closer to your goal.

I'm really happy you've made it this far. It isn't easy doing this and sometimes it's not fun either. I say sometimes, but for some people it's never fun. I was one of those, but eventually working out became a habit that made me feel bad when I skipped it. So get that fitness fix and let's get right into the exercise routines.

This chapter gives you the exercises needed for weeks 5 and 6. If you're ready to move forward, then continue with the training program below.

Week 5 Mud Race Training

Monday Training Routine (Week 5)
Warm-up Routine
(do each exercise in order for 1 minute):
- Jog in place
- Jumping Jacks
- Lunge Walks
- Arm Circles

Exercise Routine:
- Squats - 4x 30 reps
- Lateral Hops*- 5x 30 seconds
- Mountain Climbers* - 5x 40 seconds

Do back to back before resting.

Tuesday Training Routine (Week 5)
Warm-up Routine
(do each exercise in order for 1 minute):
- Jog in place
- Jumping Jacks
- Lunge Walks

- Arm Circles

Exercise Routine:
- Push-ups - 4x 15-20 reps
- Bear Crawls - 3x 30 Yards
- Bent over Rows - 4x 15-20 reps

Wednesday Training Routine (Week 5)
Find a nice walking trail and walk / jog 5 miles today.

Thursday Training Routine (Week 5)
Warm-up Routine
(do each exercise in order for 1 minute):
- Jog in place
- Jumping Jacks
- Lunge Walks
- Arm Circles

Exercise Routine:
- Pull-ups - 4x 10 reps
- Squats - 3x 40 reps
- Burpees* - 4x 20 reps

- Lateral Hops* - 4x 30 seconds

Do burpees and lateral hops back to back

Friday Training Routine (Week 5)
Warm-up Routine
(do each exercise in order for 1 minute):
- Jog in place
- Jumping Jacks
- Lunge Walks
- Arm Circles

Exercise Routine:
- Chair Dips - 4x 15-20 reps
- Squats - 3x 40 reps
- Bear Crawls* - 4x 20 yards
- Sprints* - 4x 20 seconds

Do bear crawls and sprints back to back before resting

Saturday Training Routine (Week 5)
Burpee run Time! That's right, do a 3 mile burpee run.

Sunday Training Routine (Week 5)
Just take a chill pill and relax.

Week 6 Mud Race Training

Monday Training Routine (Week 6)
Warm-up Routine
(do each exercise in order for 1 minute):
- Jog in place
- Jumping Jacks
- Lunge Walks
- Arm Circles

Exercise Routine:
- Pull-ups - 4x 12 reps
- Squats - 3x 40 reps
- Burpees* - 4x 20 reps
- Lateral Hops* - 4x 30 seconds

Do burpees and lateral back to back.

Tuesday Training Routine (Week 6)
Warm-up Routine
(do each exercise in order for 1 minute):
- Jog in place
- Jumping Jacks

- Lunge Walks
- Arm Circles

Exercise Routine:
- Push-ups - 4x 15-20 reps
- Bear Crawls* - 4x 20 yards
- Sprints* - 4x 20 seconds

Do back to back before resting.

Wednesday Training Routine (Week 6)
Find a nice walking trail and walk / jog 5 miles today.

Thursday Training Routine (Week 6)
Warm-up Routine
(do each exercise in order for 1 minute)
- Jog in place
- Jumping Jacks
- Lunge Walks
- Arm Circles

Exercise Routine:
- Pull-ups - 4x 12 reps
- Squats - 3x 40 reps

- Mountain Climbers* - 4x 20 seconds
- Lateral Hops* - 4x 30 seconds

Do back to back before resting.

Friday Training Routine (Week 6)
Warm-up Routine

(do each exercise in order for 1 minute)
- Jog in place
- Jumping Jacks
- Lunge Walks
- Arm Circles

Exercise Routine:
- Push-ups - 4x 15-20 reps
- Chair Dips - 4x 15-20 reps
- Burpees* - 4x 20 reps
- Bear Crawls* - 4x 15-20 reps

Do back to back before resting.

Saturday Training Routine (Week 6)

Another great burpee run! Go 3 miles on a burpee run.

Sunday Training Routine (Week 6)
Relax and take some time for yourself.

That's it for weeks 5 and 6. Next, we'll finish the training program and start working towards what to expect on Race Day. If you've had to skip a day or two here and there, that's fine, but try to keep being consistent and working towards the goal. You're almost there!

CHAPTER 6
WEEK 7 & 8

The time has come! After 6 weeks of preparation, the last two weeks of mud race training has arrived. Now is the time where your training comes full circle. Now is the time where you should start to realize how far you have come. If you've been consistent on this mud run training regimen, you

should've gained some or all of the following health benefits:
- Increased muscular strength
- Increased muscle mass
- Increased energy levels
- Increased endurance levels
- Reduction of body fat % (i.e., weight loss)
- Feeling quicker and lighter on your feet

If you experienced at least one of those health benefits, you have enhanced your ability to do well at the mud race. You need to finish strong these next two weeks. So without further ado, here are the week 7 and 8 training schedules.

Week 7 Mud Race Training

Monday Training Routine (Week 7)
Warm-up Routine
(do each exercise in order for 1 minute):

- Jog in place
- Jumping Jacks
- Lunge Walks
- Arm Circles

Exercise Routine:
- Pull-ups - 4x 12 reps
- Run up a hill - 6x 30 seconds
- Mountain Climbers* - 5x 30 seconds
- Lateral Hops* - 5x 30 seconds

Do back to back before resting.

Tuesday Training Routine (Week 7)
Warm-up Routine
(do each exercise in order for 1 minute):
- Jog in place
- Jumping Jacks
- Lunge Walks
- Arm Circles

Exercise Routine:
- Push-ups - 4x 15-20 reps
- Squats - 6x 30 reps

- Bent over rows - 5x 15-20 reps
- Burpees   4x 30 reps

Wednesday Training Routine (Week 7)
Take a 5 mile walk / jog.

Thursday Training Routine (Week 7)
Warm-up Routine
(do each exercise in order for 1 minute):
- Jog in place
- Jumping Jacks
- Lunge Walks
- Arm Circles

Exercise Routine
(Super Cardio time!):
- Mountain Climbers - 5x 30 seconds
- Lateral Hops - 5x 30 seconds
- Run up a hill - 6x 30 seconds
- Bear Crawls - 5x 20 yards
- Sprints - 5x 30 seconds

Friday Training Routine (Week 7)

Warm-up Routine

(do each exercise in order for 1 minute):
- Jog in place
- Jumping Jacks
- Lunge Walks
- Arm Circles

Exercise Routine:
- Pull-ups - 4x 12 reps
- Run up a hill - 6x 30 seconds
- Mountain Climbers* - 5x 30 seconds
- Lateral Hops* - 5x 30 seconds

Do back to back before resting.

Saturday Training Routine (Week 7)

Burpee run! Do a 4 mile burpee run.

Sunday Training Routine (Week 7)

Catch up on your favorite shows or read a book. Just relax.

Week 8 Mud Race Training

Monday Training Routine (Week 8)
Warm-up Routine
(do each exercise in order for 1 minute):
- Jog in place
- Jumping Jacks
- Lunge Walks
- Arm Circles

Exercise Routine
(Super Cardio time!):
- Mountain Climbers - 5x 30 seconds
- Lateral Hops - 5x 30 seconds
- Run up a hill - 6x 30 seconds
- Bear Crawls - 5x 20 yards
- Sprints - 5x 30 seconds

Tuesday Training Routine (Week 8)
Warm-up Routine
(do each exercise in order for 1 minute):
- Jog in place
- Jumping Jacks

- Lunge Walks
- Arm Circles

Exercise Routine:
- Push-ups - 5x 15-20 reps
- Squats - 6x 30 reps
- Bent over rows - 5x 15-20 reps
- Burpees - 5x 30 reps

Wednesday Training Routine (Week 8)
Walk / Jog for 5 miles.

Thursday 8 Training Routine (Week 8)
Warm-up Routine
(do each exercise in order for 1 minute):
- Jog in place
- Jumping Jacks
- Lunge Walks
- Arm Circles

Exercise Routine:
- Pull-ups - 4x 12 reps
- Run up a hill - 6x 30 seconds

- Mountain Climbers* - 5x 30 seconds
- Lateral Hops* - 5x 30 seconds

Do lateral hops and mountain climbers back to back

Friday Training Routine (Week 8)

Rest up for the race.

Saturday Training Routine (Week 8)

Race Day (or maybe Sunday)!

Sunday Training Routine (Week 8)

Spend quality time with your family and friends. You just completed something pretty amazing.

Regardless of what type of mud race you're competing in, if you successfully completed this eight week mud run training guide, you should be fully prepared to handle it.

Another note: please make sure you consult a doctor before starting this or any other training program.

Hopefully, through all the tough training, you enjoyed the journey of getting in better shape to compete in the mud run.

CHAPTER 7
Race Day

You've made it... well, almost. It's race day! Let's back up a little. Before race day you need to do a little preparation. Here are some of the things you'll need to bring with you.

Sunscreen

Whether it's going to be hot or cold, you're still going to be outside for an extended amount of time getting exposed to those awful UV rays. Wear your sunscreen.

Knee braces

This is truly optional. I tore my ACL in 2001 and have worn knee braces at every mud run I've run in since. Most people don't wear them, but I recommend them if you've had knee issues in the past.

Clothes

Wear old cloths that you're prepared to throw away. It's very likely that you won't get all the mud out. That's fine. They give you a new shirt afterwards anyway☺. Bring a change of clothes, but be warned that they will likely get muddy, too. Don't forget to pack a change of underwear, socks, and shoes.

Towel

You'll need a towel to dry off with after the race. The usually have cold (very cold) hoses and showers to rinse the mud off of you. You won't get clean here; you'll just get some of the mud off. Again, make sure that you don't mind throwing the towel away.

Your Bag
Bring a bag to put all your stuff in. Also note that you'll likely be bringing your muddy clothes and shoes back in it. You'll either need trash bags to put those in inside your bag, or an old bag that you don't mind getting all muddy.

In that bag, be sure to have your keys and a change of clothes. You can bring your phone if you want to, but it might get stolen. I leave mine in the car.

Baby Wipes
These are fantastic. I never knew how great these where until one of my team members brought some the first time I ran in the Palmetto 200. They are excellent at cleaning junk, mud, and sweat from your face. Plus they are cool, damp, and feel amazing after a run.

Snacks and water

Bring some snacks and water for the ride home. Unless you're super lucky, you'll likely be in the car for a while getting in and out of the parking lot. I've had this turn a thirty minute drive into over an hour.

Get there early... Really early.

I recommend planning to be at the race at least an hour before your start time. That gives you time to park, get checked in, and sign your waiver. If you plan on checking a bag or changing cloths there, get there even earlier. In most cases I get to mud runs an hour and a half to two hours early just to be safe. It's fun to get there early, too. Hangout, cheer on other racers, and enjoy yourself before you get all muddy.

Also be sure to hangout afterwards to enjoy some snacks and the atmosphere. Take time to cheer on fellow racers and marvel in your accomplishments. Good luck!

CHAPTER 8
NUTRITION

Getting through several weeks of grueling, high-intense training is 50% of what it takes to be mud run ready. The other 50% is consuming proper foods and beverages, and following the other helpful tips below.

Drink at least half of your bodyweight in water ounces.

It is nearly impossible to fully function

without drinking water. Since our body is made up of about 70% water, it makes sense to drink an adequate amount of it per day. While it has numerous benefits, the main benefit of drinking water is it helps cleanse your system, which makes it easier for your body to do things such as burn fat. If you know that weight loss would help your preparation efforts for the mud race, then start drinking more water. At least aim to drink half of your bodyweight in ounces. For instance, if you weigh 180 pounds, then drink about 90 ounces of water per day. **Note: Please drink water before, during, and after your mud run and all training activities, especially if you're competing in a hot climate**. Getting dehydrated on race day is not what you want.

Eat an adequate amount of slow-digesting carbs per day.

While carbs may get a bad rep in most of today's fad diet books, you need slow-digesting carbs to have energy to run through your training days. Here is the list of slow-digesting carbs:

- Fresh fruit (apples, oranges, grapes, etc.)
- Non-starchy vegetables (spinach, kale, tomatoes, broccoli, cauliflower, cucumber onions, asparagus, carrots, mushrooms, etc.)
- Sweet potatoes
- Nuts (walnuts, macadamia nuts, pecans, etc.)
- Natural nut butter
- Steel-cut oats

Slow-digesting carbs are perfect to eat before every mud run training session and the day of the race. Unlike fast-digesting carbs (candy, cookies, sugars, etc.), they provide a steady dose of carbs throughout the day that will help maintain high energy levels, i.e. no crash.

Aim for at least 3 to 4 servings of milk per week.

Got milk? I'm sure you know that milk supports strong, healthy bones, which will improve injury prevention while running. Not only that, but milk aids in weight loss. In a research study, people who ate a reduced-calorie diet that was rich in dairy (including milk) lost more weight than those who ate a diet low in dairy. So if you need to lose weight and build strong leg muscles before race day, milk will do your body good.

Don't compare yourself to other runners.

The last thing you want to do is try to compare yourself to others who have been running 5k races for years. As a newbie, you simply need to focus on doing YOUR best. You can't expect to be the best racer at your first race. Michael Jordan wasn't considered the greatest basketball player as a rookie. He had to earn that title by putting in consistent, high-quality effort throughout his career. If you expect to be the best (or one of the best) mud run racer, be prepared to continually put your best effort into your training. Or, if you're like me, just enjoy watching the elites run and be happy that you are physically able to complete the race. Remember: your goal should be finishing strong, not winning.

Enjoy yourself

Through all the time that you put into preparing for and participating in this mud run, remember to enjoy yourself. Too many individuals forget that these races were created to have fun. So relax, have some fun, and do something great!

CHAPTER 9
RACE TERMS

This is a summary of the race terms that you should know before running any race. If you want to know more, read chapter two of *Surviving a 5k Race.*

5-K/8-K/10-K
The K here stands for kilometers, or 1,000 meters. A 5-K is equal to 3.1 miles; 8-K is 4.96 miles; 10-K is equal to 6.2 miles.

10-K pace

10-K pace is the time per mile (pace) that a runner will run a 10 K race (6.2 miles).

400 meters

The 400 meters is equivalent to a quarter mile or one lap around a standard track.

800 meters

The double of 400 meters as you may have already figured out is equivalent to a half-mile or two laps around a standard track.

Aerobic

Think of a jog. Aerobic is generally used to refer to running or any other form of exercise that offers a moderately paced cardiovascular workout to deliver the required amount of oxygen to your muscle tissues without allowing any appreciable buildup of lactic acid.

You can normally run at a slow aerobic pace for long periods of time, provided you have the endurance to go long distances. However, longer runs that often involve training runs are performed at an Aerobic Pace.

Anaerobic

Think of a sprint. Anaerobic is used to refer to running or other exercises that seriously gets your heart and lungs working, causing your respiratory and cardiovascular systems to deliver all or most of the oxygen required by your muscles. These exercises are fast enough that lactic acid begins to build up in your muscles, thus producing a tired, heavy feeling. Normally the pace associated with anaerobic running cannot be sustained very long.

Athena

The Athena category of runners is for weight challenged women. Typically the cutoff is set at 160 pounds (which I don't think is over weight) and normally only used for big races. I'm not a fan of these types of categories, but you'll know what it means if you see it. The purpose of the Athena category is to give runners more opportunities to win in their class.

Chip Time

Chip time refers to a technology for detecting and recording the finishing times of all the runners in a race. It's the most accurate method and can deal with the traditional problem of many runners simultaneously finishing the race as one large group. The chip time technology uses a small device that is programmed for each runner and is given to the runner when they check in for the race. These miniature devices can be as small as an inconspicuous bracelet or slightly larger. The chip, which is generally attached to your shoe laces or worn around your arm, sends a signal to another device that's typically hidden under a strip of rubber or carpet at the start and finish lines of the race. It automatically records your exact time at the end of the race. Usually you are asked to return the chip in to the race organizers after you finish.

Clydesdale
The Clydesdale category of runners is for weight challenged men. Typically the cutoff is set at 220 pounds (which I don't think is over weight) and normally only used for big races. I'm not a fan of these types of categories, but you'll know what it means if you see it. The purpose is to give runners more opportunities to win in their class.

Cool-down
Slow running, jogging, or even brisk walking done after a workout to loosen muscles and rid the body of lactic acid.

CR
Course record.

Cushioning (Shock Absorption)
It's the ability of a shoe to absorb the impact

of your foot striking the ground.

DNF
Did not finish.

DNS
Did not start.

DOMS (Delayed Onset Muscle Soreness)
A type of muscle soreness that normally peaks about 48 hours after an intense workout or run.

Elite Runner
A runner who is ubber fast and has reached the highest level in his sport.

Fartlek (Intervals)
Sometimes called intervals. A fartlek is a variable pace running technique which includes a mixture of slow running, running at a moderate speed, and short, fast sprints. Fartlek training is a way to increase speed and endurance. I've found it's great for

runners just starting to add distance. I would recommend intervals after building a 5K base when trying to increase your distance or your speed.

"Hitting the Wall"
The point in a race when your muscles become depleted and a feeling of fatigue hits you. It's when you feel like you can't run anymore. I "hit the wall" during the 2007 OBX Marathon on mile 22. It's rough.

Junk Miles
In my opinion, and for this book, there is no such thing. Some more experienced runners will say that junk miles are runs at an easy pace put into a training program so that you can reach a weekly or monthly mileage total. They often serve as recovery from harder, more intense workouts. I believe that all miles count and help you, especially when you're just starting running or working to complete your first 5 or 10K.

Lactic Acid

A substance which forms in your muscles as a result of the breakdown of glucose. Lactic acid is associated with muscle soreness and muscle fatigue.

LSD

A popular hallucinogen from the 70s... just kidding. LSD stands for "Long, Slow Distance," which refers to longer, easier (slower paced) training runs. These runs can help when training for races, both long and short. For example, an LSD for a 7 minute per mile 5K racer might be a 9 minute 5-miler LSD.

Marathon

A 26.2 mile race. This race got its name in 490 B.C. when a Greek soldier name Philippides ran the distance from the battle of Marathon to Athens. The distance was supposedly 26.2 miles.

Master

Also called a Veteran. A Master is a runner over the age of 40.

Maximum Heart Rate
The maximum heart rate achieved during a specified workout.

"Metric Mile"
This used to confuse the crap out of me, but basically it's just 1500 meters. It's the international distance closest to the imperial mile used in racing.

Mile
I hope you know what a mile is, but if you don't its 1609 meters, 5280 feet, or 1760 yards.

Negative Splits
Running the second half of a race faster than the first half, or more specifically, running later miles faster than earlier miles. For example, during a 5K, if you might run 10 minute for your 1st mile, 9:30 for your

second, and 9 for your third.

NR
National record.

Overpronation
Usually associated with flat feet. It's where you excessively roll the foot while walking or running. Overpronation is often associated with many running injuries.

Pick-Ups
A quick burst of speed done during a run. These are normally done in shorter durations than fartleks. Pick-ups are just a way to add some excitement to what could become a boring run.

Plyometrics
Any jumping exercise. Usually highly intense and a great form of cardiovascular workout.

Pronation
Pronation is a normal and necessary motion

for walking or running. It is the inward roll of the foot as the arch of the foot collapses.

PR/PB
Personal record / personal best.

Ride
The ability of a shoe to give you a smooth transfer of a runner's weight from heel-strike to toe-off... like a car, giving you a smooth ride. A shoe's ride is a very subjective quality, but runners know it when a shoe has a good ride.

Runner's High
A feeling of bliss, joy, and well-being associated with intense running. This is apparently due to a rush of endorphins. For more on this, I highly recommend watching Robin Williams' stand-up comedy on runner's high. See more at
http://runbikehike.us/runnershigh/ .

Running Economy

This is how much oxygen your body uses when you run. When you improve your running economy, you are able to run while using a smaller amount of oxygen.

Splits
Splits refers to your times or pace at mile markers or other preplanned checkpoints along the way.

Stability
The ability of a shoe to resist excessive foot motion and hold up to stress during the run.

Strides
Strides are short, fast, and controlled runs of 50 to 150 meters. Strides can be used during training to build speed and efficiency. They can also be used to warm up before a race.

Taper
Runners usually cut back mileage (or taper down their distance) one to three weeks (depending on race distance) before a big

race. Tapering helps muscles rest so that they are ready for peak performance on race day.

Target Heart Rate
The range your heart rate reaches during aerobic training that enables you to get the most out of your workout. Your target heart rate will vary.

Tempo Runs
A type of training run where you usually run twenty to thirty minutes in length, at ten to fifteen seconds per mile slower than your 10-K race pace.

Toe Box
The front part of a shoe. A wide toe box allows plenty of room for the toes to spread.

Veteran
A term similar to a master in the U.S. According to the IAAF. Men become "veterans" on their 40th birthday and

women become "veterans" on their 35th
birthday.

Warm-up
Five to fifteen minutes of easy jogging /
walking before a race or a workout. The
purpose of a warm-up is to prevent injury
and raise your heart rate so your muscles
are looser.

WR
World record.

ABOUT THE AUTHOR

John Rouda is an IT leader, speaker, and Computer Science Professor. He currently manages a team of web developers and teaches as an adjunct faculty member at York Technical College and at Winthrop University. John currently has over 50 mobile apps in the Apple App store as well as over twenty in the Google Play Marketplace. He holds two master degrees, one in Business Administration and one in Computer Science.

He is an active runner and enjoys the challenge of mud runs. John is married to a wonderful wife and has a beautiful family that he dearly loves. You can find out more about John at http://www.johnrouda.com/ or follow him on twitter @johnrouda.

YOUR SUPPORT & MORE INFORMATION

Thanks so much for getting this book. Please understand that ratings and reviews on Amazon are the lifeblood of a book author. Getting a good review and rating helps promote this work and more work like it. To review this book, please go to http://johnrouda.com/b/r/mud/

To see more of my work, please visit my site at http://johnrouda.com/ and sign up for my newsletter. Thank you so much!

Also please note that 10% of all author royalties will be donated to charity.

25101029R00053

Printed in Great Britain
by Amazon